Reverse Aging, Disease, Weight Gain, and Energy Loss: A Guide for Women Over 50.

Adam D. Larsen

Table of contents

Chapter 1

Top 10 best anti aging food

When we eat a diet rich in colorful foods that are also high in antioxidants, good fats, water, and vital nutrients, our body will express its gratitude via the skin, which is the biggest organ. After all, the skin is often the first organ of the body to display an underlying health issue, and creams, lotions, masks, and serums can only do so much before we need to look more closely at our diets.

Even researchers have concluded that the best and safest approach to treating fine wrinkles and dull skin is by eating fruits and vegetables. Get glowing! Here are the top 10 anti-aging foods to fuel your body with for an internal glow.

1. Aquatic greens

The advantages of watercress for health are impressive. This hydrated, nutrient-rich leafy green is an excellent source of:

Vitamins A, C, K, B-1, and B-2, as well as calcium, potassium, manganese, and phosphorus.
Watercress improves circulation and mineral delivery to all body cells, which results in improved skin oxygenation. It also functions as an internal skin disinfectant. Due to its abundance of vitamins A and C, watercress may help prevent fine lines and wrinkles by neutralizing dangerous free radicals.

To try: To get beautiful skin and better health all around, throw a handful of this tasty green into your salad right now!

2. Red bell pepper

The best anti-aging antioxidants are found in abundance in red bell peppers (Reliable Source). Red bell peppers include potent antioxidants known as carotenoids in addition to their high vitamin C level, which is helpful for collagen formation.

Plant pigments called carotenoids are what give many fruits and vegetables their vivid red, yellow, and orange hues. They have several anti-inflammatory qualities. Trusted Source It may aid in preventing skin damage from the sun, pollutants in the environment, and pollution.

To try: Sliced bell peppers may be cooked in a stir-fry, added to a raw salad, or dipped in hummus as a snack.

3. Papaya

The abundance of antioxidants, vitamins, and minerals in this delectable superfood may aid to increase skin suppleness and reduce the visibility of fine lines and wrinkles. These consist of:

A, C, K, and E vitamins
calcium\spotassium
B vitamins, magnesium, phosphorus
Papaya contains a variety of antioxidants that help combat free radical damage and may even postpone the onset of aging rusted Source. Papaya also includes the enzyme papain, which is one of nature's greatest anti-inflammatory substances and offers further anti-aging properties. It may also be present in a lot of exfoliating goods.

So, sure, papaya (or products containing papain) may aid in the body's removal of dead skin cells, leaving you with luminous, youthful skin.

To try: Make a papaya mask at home for your next night in, or drizzle fresh lime juice over a huge dish of papaya for breakfast!

4. Blueberries

A and C vitamins, as well as the anti-aging antioxidant anthocyanin, are abundant in blueberries. This is what gives blueberries their stunningly rich hue of blue.

By reducing inflammation and limiting collagen loss, these potent antioxidants may be able to shield skin from damage brought on by pollution, stress, and the sun.

To try: Include this delectable fruit, which has no added sugar, in your morning smoothie or fruit bowl to boost your appearance!

5. Broccoli

Broccoli is a potent anti-inflammatory and anti-aging food full of:

nutrients C and K
different types of antioxidants
fiber\sfolate\slutein\scalcium
The key protein that provides skin its firmness and flexibility is collagen, which is produced by your body when you consume vitamin C.

To try: Broccoli may be eaten raw as a fast snack, but if you have time, lightly steam it beforehand. Cooking broccoli helps your body reap extra health advantages, from charred pieces to pesto sauces.

6. Spinach

Antioxidants included in spinach are very hydrating and aid in oxygenating and refueling the whole body. It is abundant in:

magnesium heme iron is derived from plants' vitamins A, C, E, and K lutein
The strong vitamin C concentration of this adaptable leafy green promotes the formation of collagen to maintain skin smooth and firm. That's not all, however. While vitamin K has been shown to help decrease inflammation in cells, vitamin A may assist produce healthy, lustrous hair.

To try: Include a few handfuls of spinach in a salad, smoothie, or sauté. More concepts? Check out some of our favorite spinach dishes, including cheesy burgers and spinach chips.

7. Nuts

Vitamin E, which is abundant in many nuts but notably in almonds, may aid in skin tissue healing, moisture retention, and UV protection. Furthermore, walnuts have anti-inflammatory omega-3 fatty acids from a Trusted Source, which may:

bolster skin cellular membranes
give skin a gorgeous shine by protecting its natural oil barrier and preventing sun damage.
To try: Eat a handful of mixed nuts as a snack or top your salads with them. Additionally, avoid removing the skin since studies indicate that without the skin, up to 50% of the antioxidants are lost.

8. Avocado

Fatty acids that reduce inflammation are abundant in avocados and help to maintain elastic, smooth skin. Additionally, they include a range of vital nutrients that may delay the consequences of aging, such as:

B vitamins, vitamins K, C, E, and A
potassium
Because avocados are rich in vitamin A, eating them may help us get rid of dead skin cells and reveal beautiful, glowing skin. Their carotenoid concentration may also aid in preventing skin cancer and helping to shield toxins and harm from the sun's rays.

To try: Add avocado to a salad or smoothie, or just eat it straight off the spoon. There are 23 additional ways to eat an avocado once you've tried them all. Additionally, you may use it topically as a fantastic moisturizing mask to ward against inflammation, lessen redness, and keep wrinkles at bay!

9. Sweet potatoes

Sweet potatoes get their orange hue from the antioxidant beta-carotene, which is converted to vitamin A. Skin cell turnover and the restoration of skin suppleness may be aided by vitamin ATrusted Source, which eventually results in soft, youthful-looking skin.

The vitamins C and E found in this delectable root vegetable may both shield our skin from damaging free radicals and maintain a beautiful complexion.

To try: Prepare one of these sweet potato toast dishes for an unrivaled breakfast or snack. You shouldn't just eat this vegetable on Thanksgiving!

10. Seeds of pomegranates

Pomegranates have been utilized as a fruit with therapeutic properties for millennia. Vitamin C and other powerful antioxidants are abundant. According to a reliable source, pomegranates may shield our bodies from free radical damage and lower levels of inflammation.

Punicalagins, a substance found in these beneficial fruits, may aid to protect collagen in the skin by reducing the aging process.

To try: As an anti-aging treatment, sprinkle these adorable tiny gems over a salad of baby spinach and walnuts.

Give your body an abundance of these potent nutrients.
We may give ourselves the fuel we need to look and feel our best by fueling ourselves with these anti-aging foods.

Choose colorful fruits and veggies if you want to explore more delectable plants. Richer hues often indicate better anti-radical defenses that keep your skin looking young and healthy. More colors on your plate are better, in my opinion.

It's time to delay the aging process and radiate from the inside.

Chapter 2

The reality of dieting

Diets cannot be maintained. Approximately 95% of people who try to lose weight fail, which means they start a diet but either don't succeed or, if they do, end up regaining all the weight they lost.

Diets fail because they instruct users without teaching them how to execute them. Diets often limit the kind of foods they allow and cut out whole food groupings. For instance, a low- or no-carbohydrate diet does away with carbs. Is it realistic or sustainable to believe you won't ever consume carbohydrates again? Most likely not.

Diets may at times be quite calorie-restrictive. The result is that the dieter feels bad since not eating enough causes fatigue, moodiness, and irritability.

In the end, this could encourage binge eating and other unhealthy interactions with food.

Dieting may also have negative social and cultural effects. Having to miss out on family meals during the holidays may lead to conflict and stress. Since your Thanksgiving dinner is probably not included in the "diet" you're on, you'll need to stop it to enjoy it with your family.

Diets are either "on" or "off," but life is not that way.

Last but not least, diets are only temporary, and our goal is to promote long-term, sustainable benefits. Adopt a process-driven strategy. Work on building the abilities and techniques necessary to recover from falls. While spending quality time with your family, you may choose healthful foods.

Making long-term improvement requires an attainable nutrition plan, tailored to you, pleasant, and simple to comprehend. Learn more about our strategy for coaching clients on nutrition.

Chapter 3

Disorders of eating

An eating disorder: what is it?
A variety of psychiatric illnesses called eating disorders may lead to the development of unhealthful eating patterns. They could begin with a fixation with food, their weight, or their body type.

When eating disorders are severe, they may have a substantial negative impact on health and, if ignored, can even be fatal. The second-deadliest mental disease after opiate overdose is eating disorders.

There are several symptoms that eating disorder sufferers may experience. Severe dietary restriction, eating binges, and purging actions like vomiting or excessive exercise are common symptoms.

Despite the fact that eating disorders may afflict anybody of any gender at any stage of life, they are becoming more prevalent among males and gender nonconforming individuals. These groups often report their eating problem symptoms less frequently or not at all.

What symptoms indicate an eating disorder?
Although the symptoms of various eating disorders vary, all of them include an excessive emphasis on problems with food and eating, and some of them also entail an excessive focus on weight.

It could be challenging to concentrate on other elements of life because of this obsession with food and weight.

Intense fear of weight gain or being "fat," dressing in layers to hide weight loss or stay warm, drastically limiting and restricting the amount and types of food consumed, refusing to eat certain foods, or excessive energy are just a few examples of mental and behavioral symptoms. Other signs include dramatic weight loss, concern about eating in public, obsession with weight, food, calories, fat grams, or dieting, complaints of constipation, cold intolerance, abdominal pain, lethargy, or excess energy, and excuse (in people who would typically menstruate)

Physical indicators might be:

abdominal pain and other gastrointestinal signs
unable to focus abnormal lab test findings (anemia, low thyroid levels, low hormone levels, low potassium, low blood cell counts, slow heart rate)
dizziness
fainting
experiencing constant cold
abnormalities in sleep
irregular menstrual periods

the tops of the finger joints have calluses (a sign of inducing vomiting)
thin nails and dry skin
muscular weakness with hair loss
sluggish wound healing
a compromised immune system

Why do eating disorders occur?

Numerous causes, according to experts, might be responsible for eating problems.

Genetics is one of them. People seem to be more susceptible to acquiring an eating problem if they have a sibling or parent who has one.

One last thing to consider is your personality. According to a 2015 study review, in particular, neuroticism, perfectionism, and impulsivity are three personality characteristics often connected to an increased risk of having an eating problem (Few Trusted Source).

The perceived pressure to be slim, societal desires for thinness, and media exposure that promotes these ideals are some more possible explanations (Few Trusted Source).

More recently, specialists have suggested that variations in biology and brain anatomy may possibly contribute to the development of eating disorders. Serotonin and dopamine levels, in particular, may be contributing factors.

Eating disorders types

Extreme food and weight concerns are common in a category of diseases known as eating disorders, but each disorder has its own set of symptoms and diagnostic standards. The symptoms of the six most prevalent eating disorders are listed below.

1. Binge eating disorder

Probably the most well-known eating disorder is anorexia nervosa.

It often appears throughout adolescence or early adulthood, and more women than males are typically affected (10Trusted Source).

Despite being extremely underweight, anorexics often see themselves as overweight. They often track their weight, stay away from certain meals, and drastically limit their calorie consumption.

Anorexia nervosa common signs and symptoms include:

fairly limited dietary habits
Despite being underweight, an obsession with thinness and a refusal to maintain a healthy weight are signs of great anxiety of gaining weight or persistent activities to prevent gaining weight.

a skewed body image, including the denial of being extremely underweight, and a significant impact of body weight or perceived body shape on self-esteem It's crucial to remember that identifying someone with anorexia shouldn't be primarily based on weight.

Body mass index is no longer a reliable diagnostic tool since dangers might apply to both "normal" and "overweight" individuals.

For instance, despite severe weight loss, a person with atypical anorexia may fit the criteria for anorexia yet not be underweight.

Additionally common are signs of obsessive-compulsive disorder. For instance, many anorexics are consumed with thoughts of eating all the time, and others may compulsively stockpile food or gather recipes.

Additionally, they could find it challenging to eat in public and show a strong need to control their surroundings, which limits their capacity for spontaneity.

The restricted type and the binge eating and purging type are the two varieties of anorexia that are recognized by the medical community.

People with the restricted type only diet, fast, or exercise excessively to reduce weight.

The sort of people that binge eat and then purge may consume a lot of food or very little. In both situations, individuals vomit, use laxatives or diuretics, or exercise excessively to get rid of the food they just ate.

The body may suffer significant harm from anorexia. People who have it could eventually have brittle hair and nails, frail bones, and infertility.

Anorexia, in extreme situations, may cause death via failure of the heart, brain, or several organs.

2. Binge eating disorder
Another well-known eating disorder is bulimia nervosa.

Similar to anorexia, bulimia often manifests in youth and the early stages of life and seems to affect men and women differently (From few Trusted Source).

Bulimics commonly consume abnormally large quantities of food in a short length of time.

Typically, a binge eating experience lasts until the individual feels excruciatingly full. The individual experiencing a binge often feels unable to stop eating or regulate their intake.

Although binges may occur with any kind of food, they most often happen with items that the person generally avoids.

Bulimics then make an effort to purge in order to make up for the calories they have already ingested and to feel better.

Forced vomiting, fasting, laxatives, diuretics, enemas, and strenuous exercise are examples of common purging techniques.

The symptoms of the purging or binge eating subtypes of anorexia nervosa may resemble one another rather closely. However, rather of drastically reducing their weight, bulimics typically maintain a weight that is more or less normal.

Bulimia nervosa common signs and symptoms include

instances of binge eating that occur often and leave one feeling in control
recurring instances of improper purging to avoid gaining weight
Despite having a normal weight, the worry of gaining weight prevents people from feeling confident in themselves.
An irritated and scratchy throat, swollen salivary glands, damaged tooth enamel, teeth decay, acid reflux, irritation of the intestines, severe dehydration, and hormonal imbalances are just a few bulimia side symptoms (From few Trusted Source).

Bulimia may, in extreme situations, lead to an electrolyte imbalance including sodium, potassium, and calcium. A heart attack or stroke may result from this.
3. Binge eating condition
The most frequent kind of eating problem and one of the most prevalent chronic

conditions among teenagers is binge eating disorder (From few Trusted Source).

Although it may develop later, it often starts around adolescence and the early stages of adulthood.

The signs of this illness are comparable to those of bulimia or the anorexic binge eating subtype.

For instance, they often feel out of control during bingeing and consume abnormally big quantities of food in comparatively short lengths of time.

People with binge eating disorders do not control calories or engage in purging activities to make up for their binges, such as vomiting or excessive exercise (Few Trusted Source).

According to a Few Trusted Source, common signs of binge eating disorder include:

no use of purging behaviors, such as calorie restriction, vomiting, excessive exercise, or the use of laxatives or diuretics to make up for the binge eating. eating large amounts of food quickly, in secret, and until uncomfortably full, despite not feeling hungry. feeling out of control during episodes of binge eating.
People who suffer from binge eating disorder often overeat and may not choose nutrient-dense foods. This might raise their chance of developing health issues including type 2 diabetes, heart disease, and stroke (From few Trusted Source).

4. Eating items that are not food and have no nutritional value is a symptom of the eating disorder known as pica pica.

People who suffer from pica have a need for non-food items including ice, dirt, chalk, soap, paper, hair, linen, wool, pebbles, laundry detergent, or cornstarch (From Few Trusted Source).

Pica may happen to adults, kids, and teenagers.

People with intellectual challenges, developmental disorders like autism spectrum disorder, and mental health diseases like schizophrenia are the ones who experience it the most often.

A higher risk of poisoning, infections, gastrointestinal injuries, and nutritional deficits may exist in people with pica. Pica may be lethal, depending on what you ate.

However, in order for the condition to be classified as pica, consuming non-food items must be a common practice in one's culture or religion. Additionally, a person's peers must not see it as a socially acceptable behavior.

5. Recurrent daydreaming
Another recently discovered eating problem is ruminative disorder.

It describes a situation in which a person regurgitates food that they have already digested and swallowed. They then re-chew the food and either re-swallow it or spit it out.

Usually, this ruminating starts during the first 30 minutes after a meal.

This condition may appear in a baby, child, or adult. It often develops between 3 and 12 months of age in newborns and frequently goes away on its own. Therapy is often necessary to treat the illness in both children and adults.

Rumination disorder in babies, if left untreated, may lead to severe malnutrition and weight loss, both of which are potentially deadly.

Adults suffering with this disease can limit how much they consume, particularly in public. They could lose weight as a result become underweight.

6. Restrictive/avoidant eating disorder
A long-standing condition has a new name: avoidant/restrictive food intake disorder (ARFID).

The phrase has taken the place of the diagnostic known as "feeding disease of infancy and early childhood," which was previously limited to children under the age of seven.

People who have this disease have problematic eating because they are either not interested in eating or dislike certain tastes, scents, colors, textures, or temperatures.

The following are typical signs of ARFID (from a few reliable sources):

eating habits that interfere with customary social activities, such as eating with others, weight loss or poor development for age and height nutrient deficiencies or dependence on supplements or tube feeding avoidance or restriction of food intake that prevents the person from consuming enough calories or nutrients
It's vital to remember that ARFID extends beyond typical actions like a toddler's fussy eating or an older person's reduced food intake.

Additionally, it excludes avoiding or restricting meals because of a lack of availability or because of cultural or religious customs.

What symptoms indicate an eating disorder?

The sooner you get therapy if you have an eating issue, the better your chances of healing will be. Knowing the warning signals and symptoms might assist you in determining if you need assistance.

Not everyone will exhibit each symptom at the same time, but some actions, such as (20):

actions and attitudes that suggest dieting, weight reduction, and food management are the main issues

obsession with diets, food, calories, fats, and grams

rejection of some meals

dining in public while observing other people's traditions (not allowing foods to touch, eating only particular food groups)

skipping meals or consuming little amounts of food

trendy diets or incessant dieting

strong mood swings, frequent checking of the mirror for perceived defects in looks, and intense preoccupation with body size, shape, and attractiveness

Treatment for eating disorders
Plans for treating eating disorders are individually created for each patient and may include several therapy.

Regular doctor visits and talk therapy are often part of the course of treatment.

Early treatment for eating disorders is crucial since there is a significant risk of medical consequences and suicide (From Few Trusted Source).

Some women with eating disorders in their middle years have previously battled with their weight and body image and are returning now that they have had time to heal.

However, according to Bulik, many times women are bingeing, purging, working out for hours, or undereating for the first time in their life.

It's partly because '70 is the new 50,' she explains. "It puts a lot of pressure on these ladies to maintain a physique that seems 20 years younger than it really is. That kind of puts them on this precipice, however. They begin participating in very harmful weight-control behaviors once they realize the gap between what's happening to them, their body, and the society ideal "Bulik claims.

92% of the study's participants were Caucasian, with an average age of 59.

A third of women claimed to have spent at least half of the previous five years dieting.

The research also mentioned the following other weight-control strategies:

A diet pill (7.5%)
Exercise in excess (7%).
Dialysis (2.5%)
Diuretics (2%)
(1) vomiting
1.6% of them were underweight, which is a
sign of anorexia according to their BMI.

Older bodies may be more vulnerable to
eating disorders.
Bulik believes that eating disorders may be
more harmful if they develop later in life,
albeit she lacks studies to support this.

She argues that eating disorders have a
severe impact on a person's physical health.
Aged bodies are less tenacious.

This issue is made worse by the fact that
many physicians fail to detect the signs of
eating disorders in older women or
mistakenly attribute symptoms like missed

periods to physiological changes like menopause.

There are certain stereotypes that need to be erased, she claims. "We need to alter the mental image of who receives these things."

Chapter 4

Muscle loss (Sarcopenia)

Four Elements That Hasten Muscle Loss Sarcopenia is most often brought on by age, but there are other reasons that may also induce an imbalance between muscular anabolism and catabolism.

1. Sedentary behavior, including immobility One of the main sarcopenia triggers is a lack of usage of the muscles, which causes rapid muscular deterioration and growing weakening (From Few Trusted Source).

Rapid muscle loss occurs during bed rest or immobility due to an illness or accident (From Few Trusted Source).

Two to three weeks of decreasing walking and other regular movement is also sufficient to reduce muscle mass and strength, but less noticeably (From Few Trusted Source).

Reduced activity spikes might spiral out of control. Muscle strength declines, increasing tiredness and making it harder to resume regular exercise.

2. Unhealthy Diet
Weight loss and reduced muscle mass are the outcomes of a diet with inadequate calories and protein.

Unfortunately, low-calorie and low-protein diets rise in popularity as people age because they make food taste differently, cause issues with the teeth, gums, and swallowing, or make it harder to purchase and prepare meals.

Scientists advise ingesting 25–30 grams of protein with each meal to help avoid sarcopenia (From few Trusted Source).

3. An infection

Inflammation instructs the body to break down and then repair the damaged cell groups after an accident or disease.

Inflammation that disturbs the usual balance of deconstruction and repair may also be brought on by chronic or long-term disorders, leading to muscle loss.

For instance, a study of individuals with chronic obstructive pulmonary disease (COPD)-related long-term inflammation also revealed that these individuals had reduced muscle mass.

Rheumatoid arthritis, inflammatory bowel disorders like Crohn's disease or ulcerative colitis, lupus, vasculitis, severe burns, and persistent infections like TB are a few more conditions that may induce long-term inflammation.

Blood levels of C-reactive protein, a marker of inflammation, were shown to substantially predict sarcopenia in a study of 11,249 older persons (From Few Trusted Source).

4. Excessive Stress
Additionally, a variety of additional medical disorders that put the body under greater stress are more likely to cause sarcopenia.

For instance, sarcopenia affects up to 20% of persons with chronic heart failure and those with chronic liver illness (From Few Trusted Source).

Loss of muscle occurs in chronic renal disease as a result of the body's stress and reduced exercise (From Few Trusted Source).

Sarcopenia results from the body being under a lot of stress due to cancer and its therapies (From Few Trusted Source).

Sarcopenia is one of several disorders that may manifest as a pronounced loss of strength or stamina as well as unintended weight loss. Consult your doctor if you notice any of these without a valid explanation.

Sarcopenia Can Be Reversed with Exercise

Keep your muscles active to combat sarcopenia as effectively as possible (From Few Trusted Source).

Muscle loss may be stopped or even reversed with a combination of aerobic activity, strength training, and balance training. To experience these advantages, you may need to engage in two to four weekly exercise sessions (From Few Trusted Source).

While all forms of exercise are beneficial, some are more so than others.

1. Strength Training
Weightlifting, pulling on resistance bands, or moving a body component against gravity are all examples of resistance exercise.

When you engage in resistance training, the strain on your muscles causes growth signals, which enhance your strength. Additionally, resistance training boosts the effects of hormones that promote development (From Few Trusted Source,).

By producing new proteins and activating specialized muscle stem cells known as "satellite cells," which strengthen already existing muscle, these signals work together to induce muscle cells to develop and repair themselves (From Few Trusted Source).

Resistance training is the most effective strategy to build muscle and stop it from deteriorating because of this process.

A 12-week research involving 57 seniors between the ages of 65 and 94 found that doing resistance training three times per week boosted muscular strength.

Leg presses and extending the knees against resistance on a weight machine were among the workouts used in this research (From Few Trusted Source).

2. Fitness Instruction
Sarcopenia may also be managed by consistent, heart-rate-raising activity, such as aerobic exercise and endurance training (From Few Trusted Source).

Resistance and flexibility training have also been incorporated in the majority of research on aerobic exercise for the treatment or prevention of sarcopenia as a component of a combined exercise program.

Although it is sometimes unclear whether aerobic exercise without weight training would be as effective, these combinations have repeatedly been found to prevent and reverse sarcopenia (From Few Trusted Source).

In one research, 439 women over the age of 50 were studied to determine the effects of aerobic exercise without weight training.

A five-day-per-week regimen of cycling, running, or hiking was proven to enhance muscle growth. Over the course of a year, women increased their daily participation in these activities from 15 to 45 minutes (From Few Trusted Source).

3. Strolling
Walking is an activity that most individuals can perform for free, no matter where they

live, and it can also help prevent and even reverse sarcopenia.

Six months of walking, especially for individuals with low muscle mass, boosted muscle mass, according to a study of 227 Japanese people over 65. (From Few Trusted Source).

Each participant walked a varied distance, but they were all urged to increase their daily walking by 10% on average per month.

Faster walkers were less likely to suffer sarcopenia, according to another research of 879 persons over the age of 60. (From Few Trusted Source).

Summary

The best treatment for sarcopenia is exercise. The greatest way to build muscle and strength is via resistance exercise. But walking and combined exercise regimens also combat sarcopenia.

Four Foods That Prevent Sarcopenia
You may be more susceptible to losing muscle mass if you don't consume enough calories, protein, or certain vitamins and minerals.

Even if you aren't deficient, increasing your intake of several important nutrients might help you build more muscle or get more out of your workouts.

One. Protein
Consuming protein in your diet immediately encourages the growth and strengthening of your muscular tissue.

People need to eat more protein to boost muscular development as they age because their muscles become less responsive to this signal (From Few Trusted Source).

According to one research, muscular development rose in 33 men over 70 when they took meals with at least 35 grams of protein (From Few Trusted Source).

Another research discovered that in order to promote development in a group of younger men, just 20 grams of protein were needed every meal (From Few Trusted Source).

In a third trial, seven men over the age of 65 took daily 15-gram supplementation of essential amino acids, which are the more compact protein building blocks. This led to increased muscle mass (From Few Trusted Source).

Leucine, an amino acid, plays a crucial role in controlling muscle development. Whey protein, beef, fish, eggs, and soy protein isolate are among the foods that are abundant in leucine (From Few Trusted Source).

2. Calcium

Sarcopenia and vitamin D insufficiency are associated, albeit the exact mechanisms are not well known (From Few Trusted Source).

Supplementing with vitamin D may improve muscular strength and lower the risk of falling. These advantages have not been shown in all studies, which may be because some study participants may already be receiving enough vitamin D. (From Few Trusted Source).

Uncertainty exists over the optimal vitamin D dosage for sarcopenia prevention.

Omega-3 Fatty Acids 3.

Consuming omega-3 fatty acids from seafood or supplements will promote muscle building regardless of your age (From Few Trusted Source).

A 45-woman research discovered that resistance exercise paired with a daily 2-gram fish oil supplement boosted muscular strength more than resistance training alone (From Few Trusted Source).

Omega-3 fatty acids' ability to reduce inflammation may account for some of this effect. Omega-3s, however, may also directly indicate muscle development, according to study (From Few Trusted Source).

Four. Creatine
A little protein called creatine is often produced by the liver. Although you produce enough creatine on your own to avoid being deficient, eating meat or taking a supplement may help you build more muscle.

A series of research examined the effects of daily supplementation with 5 grams of creatine on 357 people with an average age of 64.

Participants who consumed creatine saw more advantages from resistance exercise than those who did not, according to research (From Few Trusted Source).

If administered alone and without exercise, creatine is probably not helpful for sarcopenia.

SYNOPSIS: The ability of protein, vitamin D, creatine, and omega-3 fatty acids to enhance muscle development in response to exercise.

Alternate-day fasting

Regular, brief fasts are part of an eating pattern known as intermittent fasting. It is a well-liked lifestyle choice with possible advantages for wellness, illness prevention, weight reduction, and body composition.

Women may not benefit from intermittent fasting as much as men do. Women should practice modest fasting, with shorter fasts and fewer fasting days, to minimize any side effects.

Women's Health Benefits of Intermittent Fasting

In addition to helping you lose weight, intermittent fasting may also reduce your chance of contracting a variety of chronic illnesses.

Heart Health The main cause of mortality globally is heart disease (11Trusted Source).

Some of the main risk factors for the development of heart disease are high blood pressure, high LDL cholesterol, and high triglyceride levels.

In only eight weeks, intermittent fasting reduced blood pressure by 6% in one study of 16 obese men and women (2Trusted Source).

The same research discovered that intermittent fasting reduced triglycerides by 32% and LDL cholesterol by 25%. (2Trusted Source).

However, there is conflicting data linking intermittent fasting to reduced LDL cholesterol and triglyceride levels.

In a study of 40 persons of normal weight, intermittent fasting for four weeks during the Islamic holiday of Ramadan did not lower triglycerides or LDL cholesterol (12Trusted Source).

Before researchers completely comprehend the impact of intermittent fasting on heart health, higher-quality studies with more reliable methodologies are required.

Diabetes

Your risk of acquiring diabetes may be successfully managed and decreased with intermittent fasting.

Intermittent fasting seems to lessen some of the risk factors for diabetes, much like ongoing calorie restriction (3Trusted Source, 13Trusted Source, 14).

It does this primarily by decreasing insulin levels and insulin resistance (1Trusted Source, 15Trusted Source).

Six months of intermittent fasting decreased insulin levels by 29% and insulin resistance by 19% in a randomized controlled research including more than 100 overweight or obese women. The same blood sugar levels were observed (16Trusted Source).

Additionally, it has been shown that persons with pre-diabetes, a condition in which blood sugar levels are raised but not high enough to diagnose diabetes, may reduce insulin levels by 20-31% and blood sugar levels by 3-6% over the course of 8–12 weeks of intermittent fasting (3Trusted Source).

However, in terms of blood sugar, women may not benefit from intermittent fasting as much as males do.

According to a tiny research, women's blood sugar control declined after 22 days of alternate-day fasting, whereas men's blood sugar levels were unaffected (6Trusted Source).

Despite this negative impact, lowering insulin and reducing insulin resistance would probably still lower the likelihood of developing diabetes, especially in those who already have pre-diabetes.

Loss of weight
When done correctly, intermittent fasting may be a simple and efficient method of

weight loss since frequent, brief fasts can reduce your calorie intake and help you lose weight.

SUMMARY
Women who practice intermittent fasting may have weight loss and a lower risk of diabetes and heart disease. However, to validate these results, further human research are required.

For women, intermittent fasting may be done in a variety of ways. The 5:2 diet, modified alternate-day fasting, and the crescendo approach are some of the more effective strategies.

Chapter 5

Physical well-being: The value of sleep

Aging and Sleep
We often go through typical changes in our sleeping habits as we age, such as being tired sooner, waking up earlier, or getting less deep sleep. However, insomnia symptoms such as restless sleep, excessive daytime fatigue, and others are not typical aspects of aging. Your physical and mental well-being is just as vital to sleep as they were when you were younger.

A restful night's sleep strengthens memory and focus, enables your body to repair any cell damage from the previous day, and reenergizes your immune system, all of which work together to keep you healthy. Insufficient sleep in older individuals increases their risk of depression, concentration and memory issues, excessive daytime drowsiness, and overnight fall.

Inadequate sleep may also cause major health issues, such as an increased risk of diabetes, cardiovascular disease, weight issues, and breast cancer in females.

It's crucial to comprehend the underlying reasons for your sleep issues if you want to increase the quality of your sleep. You may recognize and treat age-related sleep issues, enjoy a decent night's sleep, and enhance the quality of your waking life by using the following advice.

How much sleep do elderly people require? Although everyone's needs are different, most healthy individuals need seven to nine hours of sleep per night. However, more important than a precise amount of hours is how you feel in the morning. The greatest signs that you aren't getting enough sleep include often waking up feeling exhausted or sleep-deprived.

Aging and insomnia

Tip 1: Recognize how your sleep varies as you get older.

A slow wave or deep sleep will probably decrease as you become older since your body generates less growth hormone (an especially refreshing part of the sleep cycle). When this occurs, you create less melatonin, which results in more often interrupted sleep and nighttime awakenings. As we become older, a lot of us think of ourselves as "light sleepers." You might also

Wish to sleep sooner at night and get up earlier in the morning.

To acquire the necessary amount of sleep, you either need to stay in bed later at night or make up the difference by taking a nap during the day.

Such sleep variations are often normal and don't signify a sleep issue.

issues with sleep unrelated to aging

It's typical to sometimes have sleep issues at any age. However, if you often encounter any of the following signs, you could have a sleep disorder:

Although feeling weary, you have problems falling asleep.
difficulty falling back to sleep after awakening.
After a night of sleep, you don't feel rested.
annoyance or fatigue throughout the day.
Having trouble staying awake when driving, watching television, or sitting quietly.
have trouble staying focused throughout the day.
rely on drink or sleeping drugs to go to sleep.
unable to regulate your emotions.

Tip 2: Determine the root reasons for your insomnia
The underlying yet relatively curable reasons for many occurrences of insomnia or sleep problems. All potential reasons may

be found, and the appropriate therapy can then be chosen.

Are you stressed out a lot?
Do you feel depressed? Do you feel depressed or hopeless emotionally?
Do you battle with persistent worry or anxiety?
Have you lately experienced anything traumatic?
Do you take any drugs that could be having an impact on how well you sleep?
Do you have any health issues that could keep you from sleeping?
common reasons for sleep issues and sleeplessness in elderly individuals
bad sleeping habits and conditions. These include watching TV while you sleep, drinking alcohol before bed, and having unpredictable sleep schedules. Make sure your bedroom is cozy, quiet, and dark, and that your night routines are relaxing.

medical disorders or pain. Sleep disturbances may be caused by medical illnesses such as overnight heartburn, frequent urination, pain, arthritis, asthma, diabetes, osteoporosis, and Alzheimer's disease. To handle any medical concerns, see your doctor.

Menopause and the aftermath. Many women discover that hot flashes and night sweats may make it difficult to fall asleep during menopause. Even after menopause, sleep issues might persist. Changing your daily routines may assist, particularly concerning nutrition and exercise.

Medications. The mix of medicines, as well as their negative effects, might make it difficult to fall asleep. Older folks often take more prescriptions than younger ones. To help you sleep better, your doctor could adjust the way you take your drugs.

exercise inactivity You may never feel tired or feel drowsy all the time if you have a sedentary lifestyle. Good sleep may be aided by regular aerobic activity throughout the day.

Stress. Stress may be brought on by major life changes like retiring, losing a loved one, or leaving the family home. Finding a face-to-face conversation partner is the best thing you can do for your mood.
absence of social interaction. Your activity level may be maintained and your body can be prepared for a restful night's sleep via social activities, family, and job. Try volunteering, joining a seniors' organization, or enrolling in an adult education course if you're retired.

sleep problems. Older persons are more likely to have RLS and sleep breathing disorders such as snoring and sleep apnea.

not enough sunshine. Your sleep-wake cycles and melatonin are both regulated by bright sunshine. Make an effort to spend two hours outside each day. During the day, leave the curtains open or utilize a lightbox for treatment.

Tip 3: Enhance sleeping patterns
By dealing with emotional problems, enhancing your sleeping environment, and making better choices for your everyday routine, you may often enhance your sleep. However, since every person is unique, it could take some trial and error to identify the precise adjustments that enhance your sleep the most.

Encourage a better night's sleep.
Boost your melatonin levels naturally. Artificial nighttime lighting might prevent your body from producing enough melatonin, a hormone that promotes sleep. Where it is safe to do so, use low-wattage

lights, and switch off the TV and computer at least an hour before bed.

Avoid reading at night from a backlit gadget (such as an iPad). Change to an eReader that needs an extra light source if you prefer to read from a tablet or other electronic device.

Make sure your bedroom is peaceful, cool, and dark, and that your bed is cozy. As we age, our sensitivity to noise increases and heat and light may also disrupt our sleep. It may be beneficial to use a sound machine, earplugs, or a sleep mask.

Just sleep and have sex in your bedroom. Your brain will begin to link the bedroom only with sleep and sexual activity if you avoid working, watching TV, or using your computer while in bed.

Bedroom clocks should be hidden. Your sleep may be disturbed by light, and insomnia is a certain conclusion while you are impatiently counting down the minutes.

For better sleep, follow a consistent nighttime routine.
Maintain a regular sleeping routine. Even on weekends, go to bed and get up at the same hours every day.

Silence snoring. Try using earplugs, a white noise machine, or separate bedrooms if snoring is keeping you awake.

early bedtime. Even if it means setting your bedtime earlier than usual, do it to suit how you feel.

Create relaxing bedtime routines. You may relax before bed by taking a bath, listening to music, or using a relaxation method like progressive muscle relaxation, mindfulness meditation, or deep breathing.

Limit the use of sleeping medicines and aids. Many sleep aids have adverse effects and shouldn't be used for an extended time. Sleeping drugs don't treat the underlying reasons for insomnia and, over time, may potentially make it worse.

Mix sleeping and having sex. Hugging and other forms of physical closeness, such as sex, may promote sound sleep.

Taking a nap
Sleep could provide you the energy you need to function at your best for the remainder of the day if you don't feel completely awake throughout the day. Try it out and see if it works for you.

Some advice about napping:

Keep it brief. Even five-minute naps may help with alertness and certain memory functions. Most individuals gain from keeping naps between 15 and 45 minutes.

After a prolonged snooze, you could feel drowsy and find it difficult to focus.

Sleep in. Early afternoon nap time. Your nocturnal sleep may be disturbed if you take a nap too late in the day.

Feel at ease. Try to find a quiet, comfortable space with less noise and light to snooze in.

Tip 4: To enhance sleep, use diet and exercise.

Diet and exercise are two daily behaviors that have the most impact on sleep. Along with eating a portion of food that promotes sleep throughout the day, it's crucial to pay close attention to what you put into your body in the hours before bed.

Dietary advice to enhance sleep

Avoid caffeine in the evening. Late in the day, stay away from coffee, tea, soda, and chocolate.

Don't drink alcohol just before bed. Alcohol may seem to make you tired, but it will keep you from falling asleep.

Fill up on food before going to bed. Grab a quick snack like warm milk, yogurt, or low-sugar cereal.

Limit your intake of sweets. White bread, white rice, spaghetti, and French fries are examples of foods rich in sugar and refined carbohydrates that may keep you awake at night and prevent you from entering deep, restorative sleep.

Big meals and spicy foods should be avoided just before night. Indigestion or discomfort may result from hefty or spicy meals. Try to have a little meal at least three hours before going to bed.

Reduce your beverage consumption before bed. To reduce the number of times you wake up at night to use the restroom, limit the amount of alcohol you consume one hour and a half before bed.

Exercise can help elderly folks who have sleep issues.
Your body produces molecules during exercise, particularly aerobic exercise, that help you sleep more soundly. There are a ton of things you can do even if you have mobility problems to be ready for a restful night's sleep. But before starting any new exercise regimen, always talk to your doctor.

Try:

Water or swimming workouts. Swimming laps are a mild kind of exercise that is beneficial for weak or tired muscles. Many YMCA and neighborhood pools provide water-based fitness sessions as well as swim programs specifically for senior citizens.

Dancing. If you like dancing or taking dance classes, do so. Taking dance lessons is a terrific method to increase your social circle.

pétanque, bocce, or lawn bowling. These sports with balls are a mild kind of exercise. More aerobic benefits result from walking more often and at a faster speed.

Golfing. Another activity that doesn't involve strenuous movement is golf. Spending time on the course with pals may lift your spirits and offer an aerobic boost.

Running or cycling. You can run and bike till you're old if you're in excellent form. Both exercises may be performed outside or on a treadmill or stationary bike.

Tip 5: Decrease mental tension
Sleep disruptions may also result from daytime stress and worry. When it's time to go to bed, it's crucial to learn how to let go of your thoughts and concerns.

Before you retire, keep a notebook to track your problems.

Check off things when they are accomplished, write down your objectives for tomorrow, and then cross them off your to-do list.

Play some relaxing music.

Pick out a book that relaxes you to read.

Get your lover or a friend to massage you.

To get your body ready for sleep, use relaxation techniques.

Look for occasions during the day to discuss your concerns with a friend in person.

resuming your sleep at night

It's typical to wake up more often throughout the night as you age. However, the following advice can be useful if you're having difficulties dozing off again:

Don't worry. Your body will remain awake if you worry about not being able to fall asleep again. Try to avoid thinking and instead concentrate on the emotions and physical sensations in your body.

Make unwinding a priority instead of sleeping. Without getting out of bed, try a relaxing method like deep breathing or meditation. Even if it can't replace sleep, relaxing may nevertheless help your body regenerate.

Perform a calm, unstimulating task. Get out of bed and engage in a relaxing activity, such as reading a book, if you have been awake for more than 20 minutes. But avoid screens and keep the lighting down low.

Put off your concern. If you have nighttime anxiety, write it down quickly and put off thinking about it until the next day, when it will be simpler to deal with.

Guidelines for Increasing Energy Naturally

Countless vitamins, herbs, and other products that are marketed as energy boosters may be found in stores. Even soft drinks and other meals include some of them. However, there is little to no scientific proof that supplements like chromium picolinate, ginseng, and guarana genuinely perform as energy boosters. Fortunately, you may take steps to increase your natural energy levels. Here are nine pieces of advice:

1. Manage your stress

Emotions brought on by stress use a tremendous lot of energy. Stress may be reduced by speaking with a friend or family member, joining a support group, or seeing a psychologist. Stress-reduction techniques include relaxation techniques like self-hypnosis, yoga, and tai chi.

2. Reduce your workload
Overwork is one of the primary causes of weariness. Professional, familial, and social

duties may all contribute to overwork. Make an effort to condense your list of "must-do" tasks. Determine your priorities based on the most crucial tasks. Reduce the importance of the less significant ones. If you need more assistance at work, think about asking for it.

3. Workout

Sleeping well is virtually a given when you exercise. It circulates oxygen and offers your cells extra energy to burn. Additionally, exercise may increase dopamine levels in the brain, which can improve mood. Pick up the pace sometimes when walking for further health advantages.

4. Don't smoke

Smoking endangers your health, as you are aware. However, you may not be aware that smoking drains your vitality by producing sleeplessness. Because tobacco contains nicotine, which is a stimulant, it makes it more difficult to fall asleep because it increases blood pressure, heart rate, and wakefulness-related brain waves. And if you do fall asleep, its addictive potential may start to work, rousing you from your slumber with desires.

5. Limit how much you sleep

Try getting less sleep if you believe you may be sleep deprived. This suggestion may seem strange, but figuring out how much sleep you truly need might cut down on the amount of time you spend in bed awake. In the long term, this procedure encourages longer, more restful sleep and makes it simpler to fall asleep. This is how you do it:

Don't take a snooze throughout the day.
Go to bed later than usual the first night, and only obtain four hours of sleep.
If you believe you slept well during those four hours, extend your sleep the next night by an additional 15 to 30 minutes.

Continue increasing sleep each night as long as you're getting quality rest the whole time you're in bed.

6. Fuel up on food

You may be able to prevent the energy slump that often follows the consumption of rapidly absorbed sweets or refined carbohydrates by choosing to consume foods with a low glycemic index, whose sugars are absorbed gradually. Whole grains, vegetables with high fiber content, nuts, and healthy oils like olive oil are foods with a low glycemic index. Foods with a high glycemic index often have higher glycemic loads. Glycemic indices for proteins and lipids are almost nil.

7. Make the most of caffeine

Having a cup of coffee may help you focus since caffeine does assist make you more aware. But you must take caffeine carefully if you want to experience its stimulating benefits. It may make you sleepy, particularly if you drink a lot of it or do so after 2 o'clock.

8. Drink in moderation

A great defense against the mid-afternoon slump is to refrain from consuming alcohol during lunch. Alcohol's sleepy effects are most noticeable around lunchtime. Similarly, if you want to have energy in the evening, stay away from a drink around five o'clock. If you're going to drink, do it in moderation and at a time when it's okay for your energy to start to fade.

9. Sip some water

What one nutrient has been demonstrated to improve performance in all endurance exercises saves the most strenuous? It is not a pricy sports beverage. It is liquid. One of the first indications that your body needs more water is weariness.

physical fitness and a willingness to adjust
5 mental adjustments
Our conscious minds are not where change takes place, and willpower is not what makes it happen. Emotions are the source of lasting transformation. Here are five mental adjustments that may help you alter your emotions and start down the path to real, long-lasting wellness.

1. identify the emotional requirements that must be satisfied.
The most important thing you could do is to be aware. to completely understand who you are, the feelings you need to be satisfied, and your ingrained patterns.

Most of us are aware of where we want to go but are unsure of how we got there. We must give ourselves some time to come to know ourselves, our motivating emotions, and how we may use them for good.

2. stop your sabotage.
Keep in mind that our emotions are directly impacted by our thoughts. That covers self-talk that is unfavorable or self-destructive. Starting down this road immediately leads us into self-defense. It means to keep and keep. Perhaps a better phrase would be to boost fat reserves while decreasing energy.

Most individuals are trying to undo two things.

Your subconscious is being impacted by these negative self-talk ideas and statements because it accepts them as real even if they are utterly ludicrous. To assist your body feel self-freedom, practice mindfulness and then swap out negative self-talk.

3. reveal past trauma.

It may be a huge tragedy, like the loss of a loved one, or it might be something smaller, like your third-grade teacher making you eat your peas. We all experience trauma, but if we repress it rather than deal with it, our body will continue to bring it up from our unconscious file cabinet, and we'll continue to act on it whether or not we're aware of it.

That is the unconscious mind's strength. We need to deal with our past trauma and let it go to make place for greater things to transform this and give our body the freedom to behave in love and positivity. Of course, this is easier said than done, and in the following weeks, we'll speak more about it.

4. Recognize the influence of decisions.

Thoughts are one thing we can control, there isn't much else in life. Our results are influenced by how we react to, perceive, and handle life's challenges.

Live in mental freedom by being conscious of your ideas and choosing to replace the bad with the good.

Pick to look for the positive in any circumstance.

5. With awareness, concentration, and repetition, rewire your brain.
The lesson to be learned is that our emotions are what cause change and the majority of our emotions are controlled by our unconscious minds. Our bodies and minds are like a deep file cabinet that might be hard to access.

You must be willing to delve deep, deal with previous trauma, and then learn to control your emotions if you want to make this transition and reprogram your mind.

You need the following three factors to bring about this paradigm shift:

Being conscious of your ingrained patterns, preferences, and the feelings they evoke.
Focus on the here and now while living in the moment to give oneself room to feel and live.
Repeating the good repeatedly and allowing yourself to experience it will help it become your mind's default pattern.

Chapter 6

A Study on Aging Psychology

It might be challenging to accept aging. There's a chance that our body won't be able to perform as well as it once could. Bones are more brittle. Aches and pains might occur often. Our eyesight deteriorates. Our hair becomes white or gray. It sometimes comes out. Our ears and nostrils swell. We get smaller.

These encounters affect us psychologically. This is particularly true in societies that don't value elders.

We have a hard time fitting in as we become older and lose value in our culture. We need to reevaluate who we are and decide on our goals. This is critical if you want to live to be a centenarian, as you'll see later in this essay.

According to estimates, 15 million older persons would need mental and behavioral health care by 2030. (APA, n.d.). Anxiety and despair might result from managing one's own or a loved one's illness. The loss of independence and loneliness are additional factors in poor mental health.

Elderly people may need assistance in managing daily tasks that they used to do on their own. Family disputes and feelings of dissatisfaction may result from this. Another fact of aging is losing a life partner.

A person may develop a mental health issue as a result of any of these circumstances as well as others.

Care for senior citizens is their area of expertise. Both private practice and healthcare institutions use them. These psychologists study how people age and develop and evaluate therapies. Their objective is to assist the older adult in resolving a difficulty and improving their wellness.

Chapter 7

Positive Theories of Aging

Let's examine the following four hypotheses from the different ones under discussion:

Theory of Disengagement
The disengagement hypothesis was created in 1961 by Elaine Cumming and William E. Henry. According to their view, as we become older, we withdraw from social roles and relationships. We act in this way because we are aware that death is near. We withdraw rather than risk having our reputation ruined by losing our talents.

Nine assumptions make up Cumming and Henry's (1961) hypothesis. As follows:

1. Everyone anticipates dying.
Older folks start to withdraw from their networks as a result of their acceptance that they are aging and losing their capacities.

2. Fewer interactions allow for more behavioral flexibility.

As a result, their conduct takes on an "I can do anything I want" attitude.

3. The experiences of men and women are different.

Men play important roles. Females don't.

4. The ego changes as it gets older.

For the younger individual to assume the position that the older adult is leaving, the older adult must move aside. The elderly person looks for their pleasure.

5. When society is prepared for it, total disengagement happens.

For older persons to transition, society must be ready for it.

6. People may get disengaged if their responsibilities are eliminated.

Roles have a gender component. Men perform work. Domestic duties are carried out by women. If they are unable to carry out their responsibilities, disengagement occurs.

7. Societal acceptance corresponds to readiness.
Society permits disengagement when an elderly person starts thinking about their mortality, feels their standing is declining and starts to lose "ego energy."

8. Relational incentives expand in a variety
Upward mobility is often one of society's incentives. The result of disengagement is horizontal rewards. People seek to fill the vertical reward deficit in their remaining interpersonal connections.

9. This hypothesis is not based on cultural context.
It adopts the cultural norms of the individual.

The whole procedure is agreeable to both the individual and society. When someone disengages depends on how valuable they are. If society still finds the individual to be helpful, disengagement is delayed.

In 1961, Cumming and Henry created and published their hypothesis. It's not current. Additionally, this hypothesis assumes that every household has a male and a female adult. Same-gender or single-parent households are not taken into account.

The Theory of Activity
According to the activity hypothesis, aging persons who participate in routine activities that they see as productive age well. It considers how important social contacts are for aging gracefully.

It was created in 1961 by Robert Havighurst and applies to all ages. When people are doing something they like, they are happy.

The Self-determination Theory of motivation is well-suited to this.

To boost intrinsic motivation, SDT emphasizes the value of autonomy, competence, and relatedness. Combining the two ideas makes it clear why a person's overall pleasure is higher.

A few people have criticized the Activity Theory (Health Research Funding, n.d.).

It begins by assuming equality. Not everyone is in the same financial or physical health situation. It's not always feasible to engage in one's preferred hobby.

Second, activities must have significance for the individual. Have you ever been given "busy work" by a teacher? Usually, you feel like you're wasting time and it's uninteresting.

Third, only earlier years are included in this approach. What happens then if you can no longer practice the area in which you have long had expertise?

Concept of Continuity
The capacity to retain one's routines, tastes, way of life, and connections as one becomes older is known as continuity theory. People strive to retain a connection between who they were and who they are becoming, according to this statement. It is comparable to the idea of crystallized intellect. One utilizes what they have learned from the past to upcoming developments.

Three layers of continuity exist. Similar to Goldilocks and the Three Bears, consider this. One is the perfect amount, while another is too much. In Continuity Theory, balance is important.

Continuity comes in two flavors as well: internal and external. While external refers to our surroundings, internal refers to our personality qualities.

Read Robert Atchley's 1998 essay, A Continuity Theory of Normal Aging, for further details.

The Perspective of the Life Course
This hypothesis takes into account both your family history and your prior life experiences. It takes a linked, proactive attitude. It covers all aspects of physical, emotional, and social development throughout a lifetime.

This idea, which was created by Glen H. Elder Jr., is based on five guiding concepts. The list below was compiled by Elder (n.d.):

Development over the lifespan: Aging and human development are ongoing processes. Agency: People create their own lives by making decisions and doing acts within the possibilities and limitations of their social and historical context.

Time and Place: The historical periods and locations that people encounter throughout their lifetimes are ingrained in and determine the direction of their lives.

Timing: Depending on when they occur in a person's life, events, and behavioral patterns have different developmental antecedents and outcomes.

10 Ideas & Techniques to Encourage Positive Aging

The five areas on earth where people live the longest are listed below. They are referred to as The Blue Zones and include Nicoya, Costa Rica; Sardinia, Italy; Loma Linda, California; and Ikaria, Greece.

According to research by Gianni Pes, Anne Herm, and Michel Poulain from 2013, Sardinia has the highest percentage of male centenarians. The Journal of Experimental Gerontology published an article on this. Dan Buettner, the creator of the Blue Zones, began to look for other "hot spots" like Sardinia.

Buettner (n.d.), working with scholars and demographers, identified nine particular lifestyle practices found in Blue Zones.

As follows:

Movement Normally
People who reside in the Blue Zones are pushed to migrate without giving it much thought. They work out by doing things like gardening.

Purpose
The Okinawans refer to this as "Ikigai," and it is the cause of your morning awakening. You'll live roughly seven more years if you find it.

Shift Down

Acquire stress management skills. In Blue Zones, people worship, think about their ancestors, relax, or enjoy happy hour.

80% Rule

Eat till you are finished. Don't eat anything extra after your smaller meal in the late afternoon or early evening. People who reside in the Blue Zones do so. They have weight management.

Plant Angle

Consume more beans. Pork is consumed by certain Blue Zones residents, although not more than a few times each month. 3–4 ounces are the serving sizes.

wine at five

Buettner found that everyone in the Blue Zones drinks alcohol, with the exception of Adventists. They have one to two glasses every day with friends and/or food. He proposes Cannonau wine from Sardinia.

Belong
The majority of the centenarians belonged to a religious group. According to their study, going to church four times each month extends your life by 4–14 years.

Family and relationships come first for persons living in the Blue Zone. Elderly parents and grandparents often reside in the same house as their offspring or close by. According to Buettner's team, this decreases the sickness and death rates of youngsters in the home.

Right Tribe Centenarians either choose or were born into their social circles. Those groups encouraged constructive conduct.
negative believes about aging
secret of anti aging
preventing illness

Interesting Age-Related Statistics

Social networking is popular among seniors. Social media is used by 64% of Americans between the ages of 50 and 64. The percentage of Americans over 65 who use social media is 37%. The most widely used platform is Facebook, with 41% of persons 65 and over visiting their pages (Pew Research Center, 2018).
For older people, volunteering is a significant aspect of life. People over 55 volunteered 3 billion hours in their communities in 2015. (Carr, 2018). Carr estimates that this is worth $77 billion.
Older female migraineurs may notice a reduction in the frequency, severity, and length of their attacks (Hassan, n.d.). Although they don't know why researchers believe it has to do with hormone shifts.
By the time they become 70, older people are 11% more emotionally stable than

Americans between the ages of 25 and 39. (Elder Options, 2018a).

Adults' intellect has been solidified with age. This indicates that they are more capable of applying their expertise to various fields than younger individuals since they have grown better at what they do (Elder Options, 2018a).

Older folks are less concerned with what others think of them (Elder Options, 2018a). Because they are the population that is increasing the quickest, older Americans have greater voting power (Elder Options, 2018a).

Those who maintain social connections as they age are healthier and happier (Elder Options, 2018b).

Perhaps older ladies have better sex lives (Thompson et al., 2011). Their research mostly included elderly postmenopausal women. Self-rated successful aging, quality of life, and sexual pleasure seem to remain steady, according to the researchers' findings (p. 1503). They studied 1235 female participants, ages 60 to 89.

At age 65, sex doesn't end. A healthy life and a healthy sex life are mutually exclusive. Older adults who are in better physical and mental health are 1.5 to 1.8 times more likely to indicate interest in having sex than those who are unwell (Lindau & Gavrilova, 2010).

As individuals become older, the quality of sex prevails over quantity (Forbes, Eaton, & Krueger, 2017). Age brings experience to the bedroom.

Did you know that the amount of times our cells may divide has a cap? It's around 50 times higher in humans. See The Science of Aging (below) for a summary of why we age and why it's OK.

Chapter 8

Negative Age-Related Beliefs

Stereotypes are "unchallenged misconceptions or inflated views" about a group, according to Dionigi (2015, p. 1). In verbal, written, and visual media, these views become ingrained. Stereotypes have an impact on how members of a group see themselves. This may be harmful or helpful.

Particularly in Western societies, aging is stigmatized in many ways. Some are unfavorable. For instance, elderly folks are sluggish and clumsy, forgetful, and unable to drive. The elderly are prone to illness. They are residents in nursing facilities. Older folks are unable to learn new things. These are a few examples.

Any words used to characterize someone above the age of 55 may be unfavorable.

They may reinforce unfavorable stereotypes. The richness of information this demographic gives is not well conveyed by terms like elderly, old, old-old, oldest-old, seniors, and the aged.

A great source is Stereotypes of Aging: Their Effects on the Health of Older Adults (Dionigi, 2015). Its primary concerns include the well-being and perceived quality of life of older persons, as well as the physical and psychological effects of stereotypes. The idea and methodology of several works in the review are explored by Dionigi (201-5).

Dionigi (2015) reveals several unsettling revelations. Among these is the notion that the prevalence of unfavorable stereotypes in Western society has an impact on older persons' cognitive and physical abilities as well as their ability to recover from illness.

The elder adult might belong to yet another underrepresented category. This makes the problem of inaccurate stereotypes worse. Dionigi's (2015) evaluation stresses the need of looking at a person's holistic health from this viewpoint, which is an essential feature.

How Does Wellbeing Define for Older Adults Change?

There isn't agreement on what constitutes well-being. Its fundamental principle is "viewing life favorably and feeling good" (CDC, n.d.). Any significant life experience might influence it either favorably or badly from this viewpoint. Age is irrelevant.

In general, cultural distinctions indicate subjective well-being (SWB). Cultural variations about a nation's prosperity and how it affects SWB are among them. According to several research, individuals in wealthy nations do not experience a greater range of emotions. When compared to those in impoverished nations, they believe they are happy, yet they are not. Personal traits influence how emotionally healthy someone is (Suh & Choi, 2018).

The way that different cultures define happiness also varies. Numerous studies contrast individualistic and collectivist societies. The former has a propensity to evaluate things from an outside, social perspective. The latter adopts a more inward-looking, individual viewpoint (Suh & Choi, 2018).

The fact that not all cultures agree on how desirable or essential happiness is making it even more difficult to define SWB. For instance, although East Asian and Islamic cultures devalue it, Western society does.

There are several perspectives on emotions and wellness. Researchers increasingly recognize the benefits of high activation positive affect in various cultures (HAP). These feelings resemble happiness and enthusiasm. In other cultures, low activation positive emotion is preferred (LAP). These qualities resemble tranquility and quiet (Suh & Choi, 2018).

The value put on the self varies among cultures. Self-esteem is a key factor in predicting happiness in Western societies. Asian cultures are not affected by this. The latter seems to cherish interpersonal harmony more (Suh & Choi, 2018).

A few factors can predict happiness at all times. Suh and Choi provide examples such as income, extraversion, and positive affect (2018).

From a broad viewpoint, the concept of SWB varies according to culture rather than age. This is one of the difficulties in coming up with a definition that is acceptable to everyone.

In the mid-to-late forties, bodily changes start to manifest themselves on a micro level. Some are little and have little impact on someone's feeling of well-being. Having to use reading glasses or bifocals, for instance.

A chronic illness, painful joints, damaged knees, or other circumstances might also have a detrimental impact. Each of these influences a person's capacity to continue participating in everyday activities.

SWB has many dimensions. In a study published in 2014, Jivraj, Nazroo, Vanhoutte, and Chandola examined life satisfaction, depressive symptoms, and overall quality of life. They sought to discover whether SWB was impacted by aging-related changes. Their results confirm that older persons have SWB that is comparable to or superior to that of younger ones. However, SWB decreases in the elderly.

According to Jivraj and colleagues (2014), elderly persons have different SWBs. Therefore, it's crucial to establish the age at which reductions in different indicators begin.

Karasawa and colleagues (2011) sought to ascertain if elderly persons in Japan and America vary from one another. Personal development, life purpose, and interpersonal well-being were the three SWB characteristics that were assessed.

Their findings revealed that both cultures scored lower for having a purpose in life. Personal development was greater among older Japanese individuals than it was among midlife adults. The reverse was true in the US. Japanese respondents had greater ratings of interpersonal well-being than Americans, although this was only true for younger individuals.

Researchers discovered gender disparities as well. In both cultures, men scored worse on interpersonal well-being. Women were more adversely affected.

They recommend including bigger sample numbers and culturally aware metrics in future research. They employed a convenience sample of 3032 Americans and 482 Japanese people for their investigation.
Age and Brain Plasticity
At age 55, neuroplasticity continues. In comparison to younger brains, the elderly brain has flexibility in a distinct region. White matter is what has changed in aging brains. The myelin-coated axons in the brain are housed in white matter. Signal transmission is sped up by myelin.

In the research by Yotsumoto and Chang (2014), older people's white matter in their brains is altered as a result of learning a new visual task. This modification was substantial. The cortex changes in younger brains.

(2013) Park and Bischof looked at how brain training affected adult learners. They were interested in finding out whether the aging brain responds differently to stimulation. They conclude from their research that participant-used methods may be to blame for variations in activation. Changes in brain activity may have pointed to neuronal plasticity, which Park and Bischof (2013) were unable to rule out.

Participating in difficult activities or receiving cognitive training may enhance cognitive performance. There is no "far-transfer" in this exercise that is just for training. The capacity to apply learning to activities with related processes is known as far transfer. The "persistence of training effects" has been praised by Park and Bischof (2013) as "outstanding."

The researchers contend that enjoyable pastimes are preferable to computer-based instruction.

Pauwels, Chalabi, and Swinnen (2018) discovered that utilizing a random practice schedule helped older persons learn tasks more effectively. They examined the abilities of young and elderly individuals to learn three different iterations of a bimanual visuomotor tracking task in their research.

They divided the subjects into groups for block training and random training. Block schedules are less demanding and more systematic.

The training was placed over three days, with follow-up occurring six days afterward. During the acquisition stage, both groups temporarily performed poorly. Contextual interference effects were to blame for this. The retention phase showed better performance from both groups.

The key message is that we can still learn complicated jobs as we become older and that we can retain our knowledge just as effectively as a younger individuals. The advantage of crystallized intellect extends to older people. This is the capacity to approach new challenges by fusing previously acquired information and experience. With age, this kind of intellect develops.

Chapter 9

Anti aging secret that turns back the clock

1. Slim Down

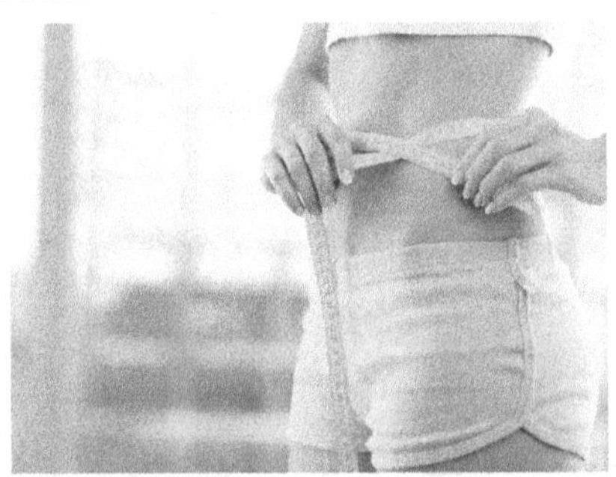

Our #1 objective every year is to lose weight, but if you reach that goal sooner rather than later, you could have more years to look forward to. Obesity and the risk of heart disease, embolisms, diabetes, and certain forms of cancer are linked, according to research published in the American Journal of Clinical Nutrition, and carrying additional pounds may instantly deplete your vitality. Thankfully, research indicates that decreasing only 10% of your body weight may have a significant impact on your life expectancy and general health.

2. Eat a banana as a snack

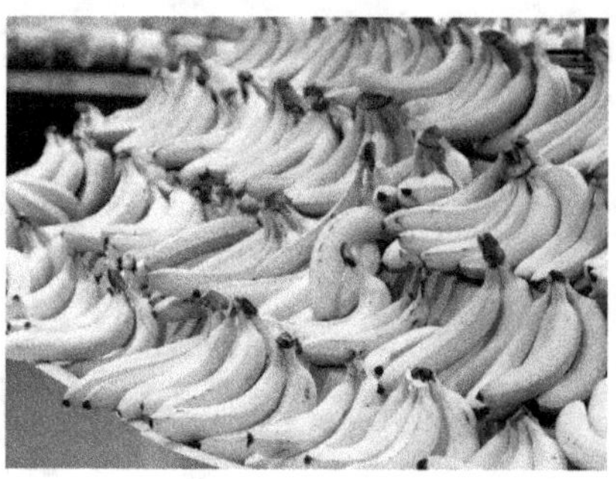

Eat a banana as a snack for a fountain of youth advice that is as simple as it is to peel. Bananas are a fantastic source of potassium, which may help maintain the health of your heart and lessen muscular cramps, making it simpler to work out consistently. Even better, Lund University researchers in Sweden have connected the resistant starch included in foods like bananas to improved gut flora, which may reduce your chance of getting Alzheimer's.

3. Include green vegetables in every meal.

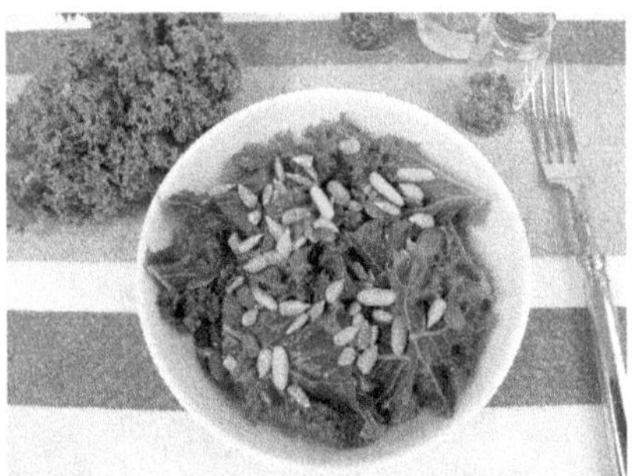

While the food pyramid suggests that grains should make up the majority of our meals, greens have the potential to keep us healthy for a longer period. Increased consumption of leafy greens is strongly connected to decreased incidence of Alzheimer's disease and other indicators of brain aging, according to research published in Alzheimer's & Dementia. The antioxidants that every cup of kale or spinach salad will bring to your meal will also greatly improve the health and brightness of your skin. Make every meal healthier by including the 40 Ingredients Nutritious Cooks Always Have in Their Kitchen on your next shopping list, in addition to all those healthy greens.

4. Eat scrambled eggs to start the day.

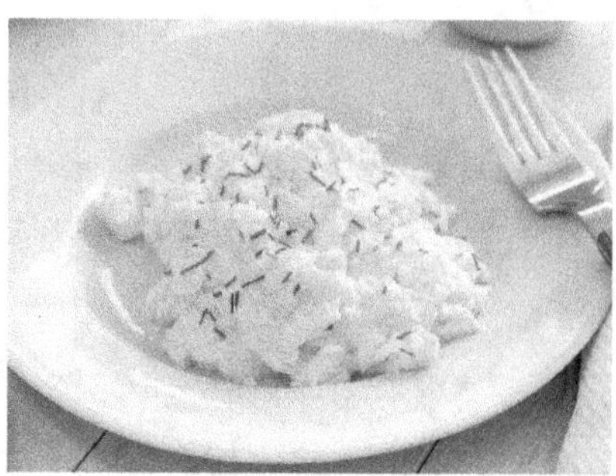

A fantastic technique to combat aging is to replace those breakfasts high in carbohydrates with some eggs. The combination of lutein and zeaxanthin, which is included in egg yolks, helps prevent macular degeneration, keeping your eyes healthy and clear as you age, according to research from the University of Wisconsin. According to a study's findings, those who ate eggs for breakfast lost considerably more weight than people who ate bagels. The study's findings were published in the International Journal of Obesity.

5. Eat a few grapes.

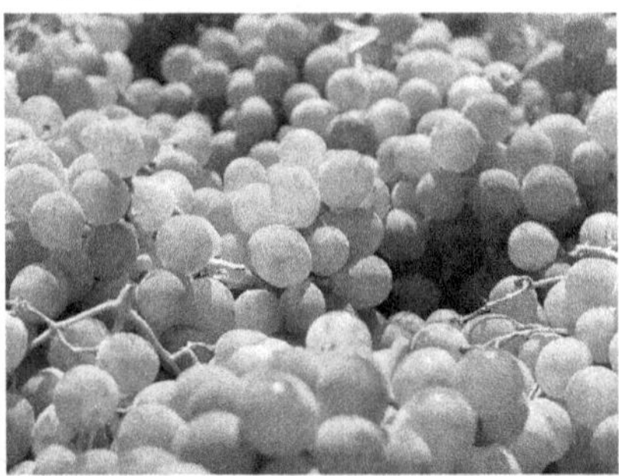

By choosing some red grapes over your typical sweet treat, you could start to feel and look younger right away. Resveratrol, which may help you fight belly fat and which research from the Washington University School of Medicine has connected to better eye circulation, keeping your eyesight sharp as you age, is abundant in red grapes.

6. Reduce Your Caloric Intake,

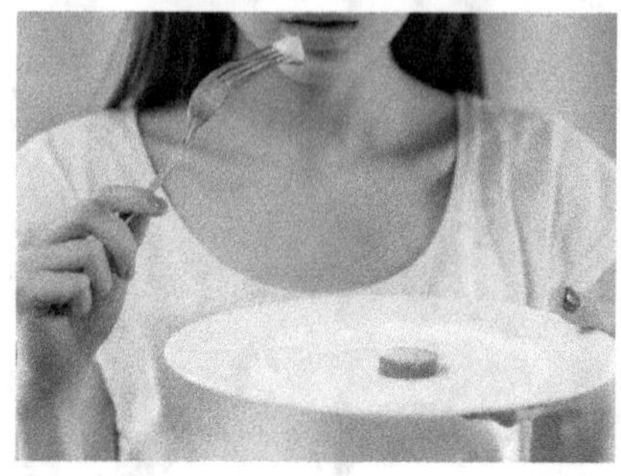

Although dieting may not always be enjoyable, it may greatly improve your health and lifespan. Not only may decreasing weight lower your chances of developing several chronic illnesses, but UCLA researchers also discovered that mice with a 65 percent caloric load reduction lived 35 to 65 percent longer than mice with relatively little caloric restriction. Additionally, they were able to lower their chance of developing tumors. The 20 Weird Reasons Why You're Gaining Weight Fast may be to blame if your attempts to lose weight are failing.

7 Eat Some Blueberries as a Snack

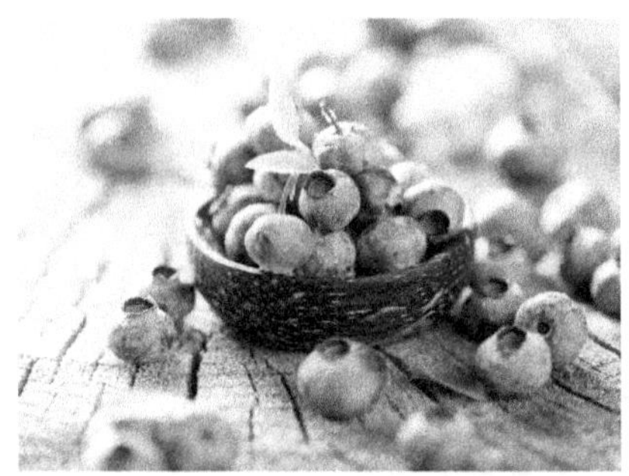

No of your age, adding some blueberries to your oatmeal or favorite smoothie will help you keep your young glow. Anthocyanins, the antioxidant pigments that give fruits like blueberries their unique color, have been shown in studies published in the Annals of the New York Academy of Sciences to considerably lower the risk of dementia in the aging brain.

8. Consider drinking black coffee.

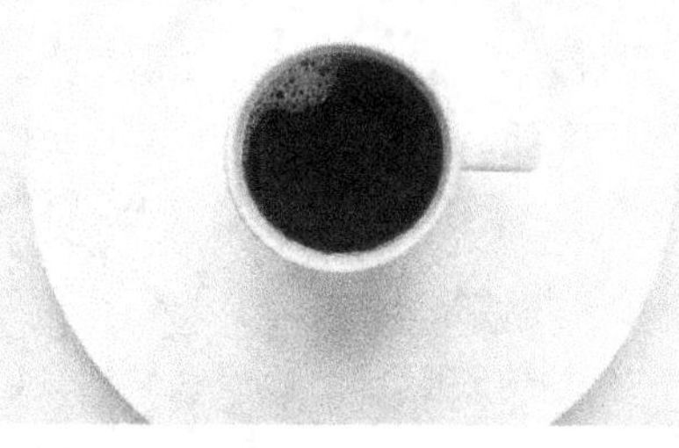

You may say goodbye to these signs of aging by simply forgoing the cream and sugar in your coffee. Dairy consumption and an elevated risk of Alzheimer's disease have been linked, according to researchers at Kyushu University, and numerous studies have linked sugar and artificial sweeteners to weight gain and an increase in belly fat, both of which can make you appear years older than you are.

9. Eat a little honey.

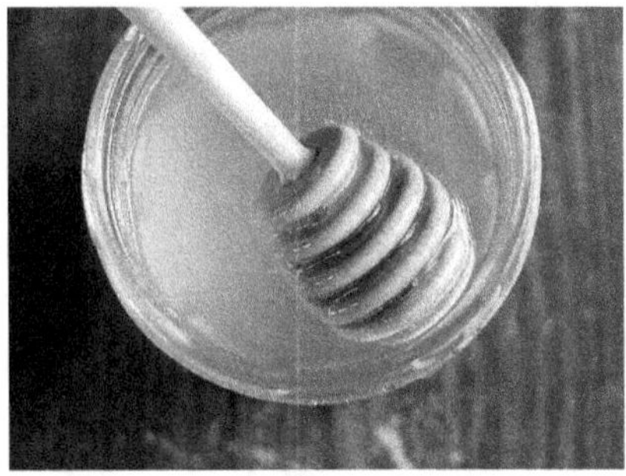

While adding a little honey to your diet may help you look and feel younger, processed sugar is not good for your health or beauty. Since honey has strong antibacterial properties, using it might help you avoid illnesses that hasten aging. By include some in your skincare regimen, you may lessen the appearance of fine lines and wrinkles while also maintaining the hydration and firmness of your skin.

10 Don't Sit All Day

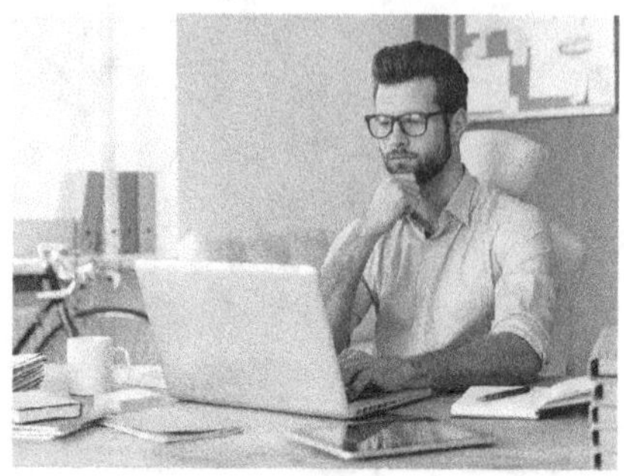

Make like Ludacris and stand up; sitting all day is hastening the aging process. Spending a lot of time on your tuchus might make you more likely to get obese and possibly pass away too soon. Even if you exercise, sitting all day may raise your chance of type 2 diabetes by up to 90% and raise your risk of sudden death significantly, according to research in the Annals of Internal Medicine. Even if you have a desk job, consider utilizing a standing desk, sitting on an exercise ball, or simply making it a point to get up and go for a walk once an hour to keep your body young and healthy.

11 Put your happiness first.

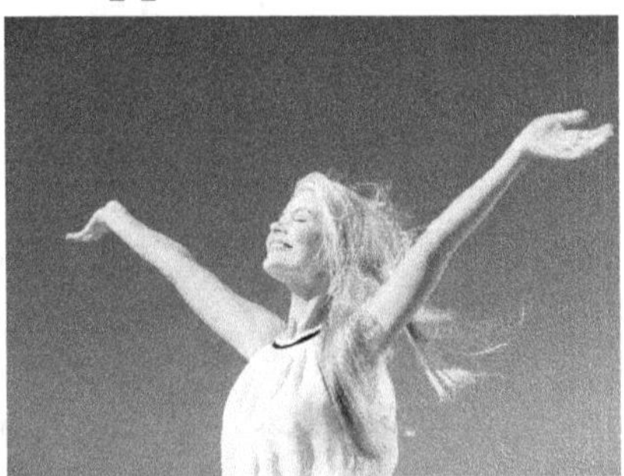

The secret to finding the fountain of youth may be found in happy individuals. A positive outlook may reduce your chance of dying young by up to 35%, according to research from University College London, and studies have shown that smiling makes you seem considerably younger than your real age.

12 Stop Eating When You're 80% Full

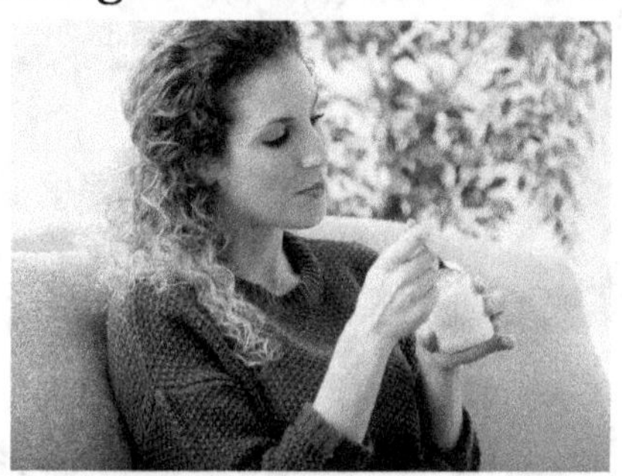

Your aging process can be sped up if you overeat at every meal. In one of the oldest communities in the world, Okinawa, Japan, residents often stopped eating when they were 80% satisfied. There are many reasons to avoid overeating when you take into account the plethora of studies that indicate calorie restriction may help slow down the aging process.

Chapter 10

Top 10 Preventive Care Examinations for People Over 50

You only have one body, therefore you should try to keep it active and functional. Age shouldn't be a reason to quit. Preventive healthcare is one of the greatest methods to keep active. Your doctor may use some screens and tests to discover issues early on before they become more serious.

Do not allow the expense of the testing to deter you. Preventive exams are covered by Medicare and the majority of health insurance. If necessary, your doctor may assist in making the case. They could also be able to refer you to programs that are free or inexpensive.

1. Check your blood pressure: Without your knowledge, high blood pressure may lead to

a heart attack, a stroke, eye difficulties, and renal problems. It's crucial to get your blood pressure tested even if you don't believe you have a problem because of this. If your blood pressure is under 120/80, it's typically okay to have a checkup at least once each year. Your doctor will likely want to check it more often if it is higher.

2. Cholesterol testing: One of the leading causes of mortality in the United States is heart disease. High cholesterol is one of the key risk factors for it. Get your cholesterol checked at least once every four to six years after turning 20. Your levels and risk for heart disease are revealed by a quick blood test.
Your chance of developing heart disease increases with age. In your 50s, it's critical to continue being tested.

3. Mammogram: The greatest method for detecting breast cancer early is, according to experts, a mammogram. On how often you

ought to get one, there is considerable disagreement.

Every woman between the ages of 50 and 74 should have a mammogram every two years, according to the U.S. Preventive Services Task Force. If you're over 40, the American Cancer Society advises getting one every year. Based on your family history and other factors, discuss the optimum timetable with your doctor.

4. Colon cancer screening: The second-leading cause of cancer-related fatalities in the United States is colon cancer. Your likelihood of receiving it increases after you age 45. Therefore, after you reach the age of fifty, your doctor will likely advise tests unless you pose an above-average risk.

Early colon cancer detection may be aided by tests. The tests you and your doctor opt to undergo and the results will determine how often you are examined. Typical screenings comprise:

Colonoscopy, typically administered every ten years

Most people get a fecal occult blood test yearly.

Most people have a sigmoidoscopy every five years, followed by a fecal occult blood test every three years.

multi-targeted stool testing for DNA alterations that may indicate a problem

X-rays are used in CT colonography to obtain images of your colon. Computer software is then used to combine the images to assist your doctor to determine if anything is amiss.

Additionally, sigmoidoscopy and colonoscopy may aid in cancer prevention. During these, your doctor could identify and remove precancerous colon polyps.

5. Pap test: This test looks for cervical cancer, which, if detected early, is manageable to treat. Even though your risk of cervical cancer declines with age, you still

require regular Pap screenings beyond menopause.

Women between the ages of 21 and 65 are advised to have a Pap test every three years by U.S. Preventive Services Task Force. If both tests are negative the first time you take them, you may elect to be tested every five years starting at age 30 using human papillomavirus (HPV) testing or a combination of the Pap and HPV tests. A Pap test could be required more often if your risk of developing cancer is greater. The ideal option for you might be suggested by your doctor.

6. Bone mineral density scan: This measures your vulnerability to osteoporosis, a bone-weakening disorder. At age 65, it is advised for all women. Your doctor could advise you to have it done sooner if you're at high risk.

Men aged 70 and older may also benefit from this check.

7. Abdominal aortic aneurysm screening: If you are a guy aged 65 to 75 who has ever smoked, experts advise getting this test. It's an ultrasound that searches for an enlarged blood artery in your belly that might burst and result in a life-threatening hemorrhage. Surgery may typically shrink swollen blood vessels. Speak with your doctor if you have a family history of this since they could suggest screening.

8. Depression screening: Although it's often disregarded, depression is a prevalent cause of adult impairment. Aging and chronic sickness might cause it to manifest. You can seek therapy for it since it's not a natural component of aging. Consult your doctor if you're experiencing sadness, hopelessness, or a lack of interest in activities you formerly found enjoyable. By having you fill out a questionnaire or respond to a few

straightforward questions, they can determine if you are depressed.

9. Diagnosis of diabetes: Over 10% of all Americans have the disease, and almost 28% of them go untreated. Diabetes with uncontrolled complications may result in limb amputation, renal failure, and blindness. Find out from your doctor how frequently you should be screened for diabetes.

10. Vaccinations: As you become older, you may need a few more shots to keep you healthy, such as:

Everyone above the age of six months old should get an annual flu vaccination.

Pneumonia vaccination: Two separate vaccine series are now advised. If you are 65 years of age or older, or if you have: